Table of Cont

MW01492025

20-0625

Healthy behavior

Eating a variety of foods, and drinking plenty of water every day.

Health terms

accurate

carbohydrate

complex carbohydrates

diet

fat

fructose

glucose

glycogen

hormone

internal organ

metabolism

minerals

nutrients

nutrition

physical activity

protein

registered dietitian

reliable

saturated fat

sucrose

trans fat

trustworthy

unsaturated fat

vitamins

Student Journal
What Are Nutrients?

Journal entry

> **Nutrition** – The study of diet —what a person eats—and health.

Write 3 things you think of when you hear the word *nutrition*.

_____

_____

_____

_____

_____

_____

_____

_____

Good sources of information about nutrition

.gov websites:

> American Dietetic Association: www.eatright.org
>
> USDA Nutrition Website: www.nutrition.gov
>
> Food and Nutrition Information Center: www.nal.usda.gov/fnic
>
> President's Council on Fitness, Sports and Nutrition: www.fitness.gov

.org websites:

> Academy of Nutrition and Dietetics: www.eatright.org
>
> American Heart Association: www.heart.org
>
> American Cancer Society: www.cancer.org

> **Nutrients** – Things we get from food that help us grow and stay alive.

© ETR **HEALTH*Smart*** Middle School

Key Nutrients for Your Body
Nutrients are the body's building blocks.
Nutrients are divided into 6 categories.

① Carbohydrates **are the main part of most human diets.** They provide the body's most important source of energy.

There are 2 types of carbohydrates:

■ Complex carbohydrates give the body lasting energy. They include starches, glycogen and some forms of fiber. At least half of your calories should come from complex carbohydrates. Whole-grain breads, cereals and pasta, as well as vegetables, fruits and beans have complex carbohydrates. Fiber comes from carbohydrates the body can't digest. It helps move waste out of the body.

■ Simple carbohydrates are sugars such as glucose, fructose and sucrose. You should limit these because they don't add a lot of vitamins and minerals to the body. They can also cause weight gain. They include foods such as fruit drinks, candy, cake and cookies.

1. What does this nutrient do for the body? _____

_____

2. What healthy foods are good sources of this nutrient? _____

_____

② Fats **include solid fats and oils.** A little fat is found in almost all foods.

The body needs a certain amount of fat to:

■ Protect against cold.

■ Provide energy for muscles.

■ Provide a layer of padding between skin and muscles.

■ Protect internal organs.

Saturated fat is solid at room temperature. It is found mainly in foods that come from animals. Too much saturated fat can cause health problems, including heart disease and cancer. Trans fats are liquid fats that have been changed to be more solid. Trans fats are found in many processed foods. They are similar to saturated fat and also cause health problems.

The healthiest sources of fat are fish, nuts and vegetable oils, which contain unsaturated fat.

1. What does this nutrient do for the body? _____

_____

2. What healthy foods are good sources of this nutrient? _____

_____

(continued)

Key Nutrients for Your Body

(continued)

③ Proteins **help make skin, muscle and bone.** They are needed to help repair damaged tissue. Too much protein doesn't build more muscles. Instead, it's burned for energy, just as carbohydrates are. About 10–30% of your calories should come from proteins. Protein is found in meat, eggs, milk and other dairy products, dried beans and nuts.

1. What does this nutrient do for the body? _____

_____

2. What healthy foods are good sources of this nutrient? _____

④ Vitamins **help control body functions such as digestion, metabolism, hormone development, wound healing and nerve function.** Vitamins help the body produce energy. Vitamins are found in all food groups, but fruits and vegetables are really good sources.

1. What does this nutrient do for the body? _____

_____

2. What healthy foods are good sources of this nutrient? _____

_____

⑤ Minerals **help with bone growth, water balance, metabolism, and nerve and muscle function.** More than 20 minerals are needed to be healthy. Common minerals include calcium, sodium, potassium, iron and zinc. Minerals are found in all food groups, but vegetables, fruits and whole grains are good sources.

1. What does this nutrient do for the body? _____

_____

2. What healthy foods are good sources of this nutrient? _____

⑥ Water **makes up 50–75% of your body weight.** Water is so important that your body can't live for more than a few days without it.

Water has many functions, such as helping to carry nutrients and oxygen throughout the body and helping in digestion. Your body loses water every day through sweating, breathing and urinating (peeing). So it's important to drink enough water every day.

1. What does this nutrient do for the body? _____

_____

2. What healthy foods are good sources of this nutrient? _____

What I Know About Nutrients

Directions: Match the nutrient to its main function in the body. Then answer the questions based on what you've learned about nutrients.

_____ Carbohydrates

_____ Fats

_____ Proteins

_____ Vitamins

_____ Minerals

_____ Water

A. Make skin, muscle and bone, and repair damaged tissue.

B. Control body processes, including digestion, healing and energy production.

C. Insulate against cold and protect internal organs.

D. Provide the body's most important source of energy.

E. Carries nutrients and oxygen throughout the body.

F. Contribute to water balance, metabolism, and nerve and muscle function.

1 **What are 2 foods that give you each of these nutrients?**

Complex carbohydrates:

1. _____

2. _____

Protein:

1. _____

2. _____

Healthy fats:

1. _____

2. _____

Vitamins:

1. _____

2. _____

Minerals:

1. _____

2. _____

2 **Why is it important to drink plenty of water?**

_____

_____

_____

_____

_____

_____

Self-Check
- ☐ I matched each nutrient to its function.
- ☐ I answered the questions clearly using what I learned about nutrients.

Healthy behavior

Eating a variety of foods and the right number of servings from each food group every day.

Health terms

diet

food group

recommended

serving

Student Journal
What Should I Eat & How Much?

Journal entry

Draw a picture of a favorite meal. Try to show how much you usually eat of each food item in this meal.

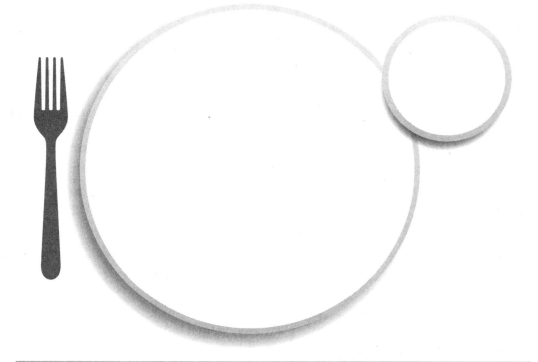

MyPlate

How does your meal compare to MyPlate?

_____

_____

_____

_____

_____

_____

_____

_____

MyPlate for Teens

Fruits give your body complex carbohydrates, vitamins, minerals and fiber.

1. _____

2. _____

Grains give your body complex carbohydrates, vitamins, minerals and fiber. At least half the grains you choose each day should be whole grains. Whole grains are the grains that contain all parts of the grain kernel.

1. _____

2. _____

Dairy gives your body protein, vitamins and minerals.

1. _____

2. _____

Vegetables give your body complex carbohydrates, vitamins, minerals and fiber.

1. _____

2. _____

Protein gives your body protein, vitamins and minerals.

1. _____

2. _____

How Much Should I Eat?

Grains You need **5–10 ounces** a day.

These all count as 1 ounce of grains:

- 1 slice bread
- ½ hot dog bun or hamburger bun
- ½ small bagel
- ½ English muffin
- 5 whole-wheat crackers
- 6-inch tortilla
- 1 cup cold cereal
- ½ cup cooked cereal
- ½ cup cooked rice
- ½ cup cooked pasta

2 whole-grain foods I like to eat:

1. _____

2. _____

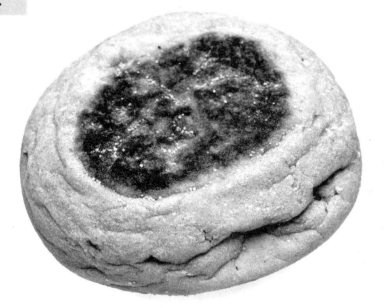

This is **1 whole** English muffin.
It counts as **2 ounces** of grains.

Vegetables You need **2–4 cups** a day.

These all count as ½ cup of vegetables:

- ½ cup cooked vegetables
- ½ cup raw chopped vegetables
- 1 cup raw leafy vegetables
- ½ cup vegetable juice
- ½ medium baked potato
- ½ cup mashed potatoes
- ½ cup tomato sauce

2 vegetables I like to eat:

1. _____

2. _____

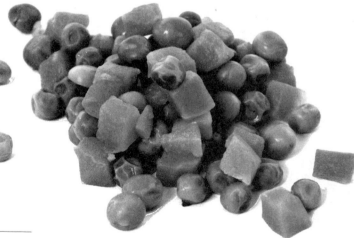

This is **½ cup** of cooked vegetables.

(continued)

© ETR **HEALTH*Smart*** Middle School

How Much Should I Eat? (continued)

Fruits You need 1½–2½ cups a day.

These all count as ½ cup of fruit:

- 1 small fruit (apple, orange, pear, peach)
- ½ cup of berries
- ¼ cup dried fruit
- ½ cup canned fruit
- ½ cup 100% fruit juice

2 fruits I like to eat:

1. _____
2. _____

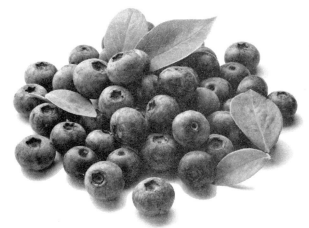

This is ½ **cup** of berries.

Dairy You need 3 cups a day.

These all count as 1 cup of dairy:

- 1 cup (8 ounces) milk or yogurt
- 1½ ounces cheese (or 2 slices)
- 2 cups cottage cheese
- 1 cup frozen yogurt
- 1 cup calcium–fortified soymilk

2 dairy foods I like to eat:

1. _____
2. _____

This is **1½ ounces** of cheese.
It counts as **1 cup** of dairy.

Protein You need 5–7 ounces a day.

These all count as 1 ounce of protein:

- 1 ounce cooked lean meat, poultry or fish (a small hamburger patty is about 3 ounces)
- 1 egg
- ¼ cup tofu
- ¼ cup cooked beans or peas
- 1 tablespoon peanut butter
- ½ ounce nuts or seeds (12 almonds)

2 protein foods I like to eat:

1. _____
2. _____

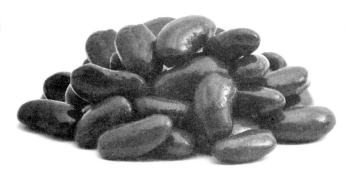

This is ½ **cup** of cooked beans.
It counts as **2 ounces** of protein.

Filling MyPlate

Directions: For each food group, name the main nutrient(s) it provides, tell how much to eat each day, and list at least 3 examples of healthy foods from that food group. Then answer the questions.

What nutrient(s) does this group provide?

_____

How much should you eat each day?

_____

Healthy food examples:

What nutrient(s) does this group provide?

_____

How much should you eat each day?

_____

Healthy food examples:

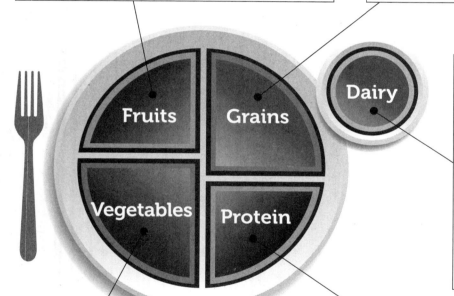

What nutrient(s) does this group provide?

_____

_____

How much should you eat each day?

_____

Healthy food examples:

What nutrient(s) does this group provide?

_____

How much should you eat each day?

_____

Healthy food examples:

What nutrient(s) does this group provide?

_____

How much should you eat each day?

_____

Healthy food examples:

(continued)

© ETR   **HEALTH***Smart* Middle School

Filling MyPlate (continued)

Questions

① Why do teens need to eat more from the grains, fruits and vegetables food groups?

_____

_____

_____

_____

_____

_____

_____

② Why do teens not need to eat as much from the protein food group?

_____

_____

_____

_____

_____

_____

_____

_____

③ What are at least 3 foods that provide fiber?

1. _____

2. _____

3. _____

Self-Check

☐ I named the main nutrient(s) in each food group.

☐ I listed the daily amount for each food group.

☐ I identified at least 3 healthy choices from each food group.

☐ I answered the questions clearly and completely.

Healthy behavior

Eating lots of fruits, vegetables and whole-grain products, and eating less unhealthy fat, added sugar and salt.

Health terms

analyze

fiber

guidelines

high blood pressure

moderation

nutritionist

processed foods

refined grain

registered dietitian

saturated fat

sodium

trans fat

vitamins

Student Journal
Assessing My Eating Habits

Journal entry

Draw or describe what you had for dinner or supper last night.

Use what you've learned about MyPlate to look at your meal. What is one way you could improve to eat healthier?

_____

_____

_____

_____

_____

(continued)

© ETR **HEALTH** *Smart* Middle School

Student Journal
Assessing My Eating Habits (continued)

Guidelines for healthy eating

1. Make half your plate fruits and vegetables.

2. Make at least half your grains whole grains.

3. Eat less unhealthy fat.

4. Eat less added sugar.

5. Eat less salt.

6. Vary your protein routine.

Eating in moderation

What does "eating in moderation" mean?

_____

_____

_____

_____

What are the benefits of eating in moderation?

_____

_____

_____

_____

My additional notes

_____

_____

_____

_____

_____

Assessing My Eating Habits

> **Directions:** Read each guideline and rate yourself. Then describe one way you could improve your eating habits in this area and answer the question.

▶ Guideline 1

Make half your plate fruits and vegetables.

Fruits and vegetables should be key parts of your daily diet. Fruits and vegetables provide vitamins, minerals, complex carbohydrates and fiber important for good health.

How I'm Doing	One Way I Can Improve
Rate yourself on eating enough fruits and vegetables daily. ☐ **Excellent:** I eat at least 1½–2½ cups of fruit and 2–4 cups of vegetables daily. ☐ **Good:** I eat 1 cup of fruit and 1–2 cups of vegetables daily. ☐ **Fair:** I eat ½ cup of fruit and ½–1 cup of vegetables every day. ☐ **Poor:** I rarely eat fruits and vegetables.	

▶ Guideline 2

Make at least half your grains whole grains.

Whole-grain foods include whole-grain bread, oatmeal, cereal and pasta. These foods provide vitamins, minerals and carbohydrates.

Whole-grain foods provide more nutrients than refined-grain foods.

Refined-grain foods include many crackers, cookies, white breads, cake and other foods high in fat and sugar. Choose these less often.

How I'm Doing	One Way I Can Improve
Rate yourself on eating the right amount of grains daily, especially whole grains. ☐ **Excellent:** I eat 5–10 oz. of grains daily—at least half are whole grain. ☐ **Good:** I eat 5–10 oz. of grains daily—some are whole grain. ☐ **Fair:** I eat 1–4 oz. of grains daily—some are whole grain. ☐ **Poor:** I rarely eat whole-grain foods. 1 ounce of grain is equal to 1 piece of bread, 1 cup of cereal, or ½ cup cooked rice or pasta.	

(continued)

© ETR   **HEALTH**Smart Middle School

Assessing My Eating Habits (continued)

▶ Guideline 3

Eat less unhealthy fat.

Teens should get no more than 25–35% of the calories they eat from fat. Get most of your fat from healthy sources such as fish, nuts and vegetable oils. Limit french fries, hamburgers, chips, chocolate and pizza. These foods usually have high amounts of saturated fat and lots of calories. Try to avoid trans fats.

How I'm Doing	One Way I Can Improve
Rate yourself on eating a diet low in unhealthy fat. ☐ **Excellent:** I eat about the right amount of fat from healthy sources. ☐ **Good:** I eat a little too much fat, but usually choose healthy sources. ☐ **Fair:** I eat too much fat from unhealthy sources. ☐ **Poor:** I eat way too much fat from unhealthy sources.	

▶ Guideline 4

Eat less added sugar.

Fruits, honey and some vegetables naturally contain sugar. But when sugar is added to foods, it contributes to weight gain, tooth decay and some types of diseases.

How I'm Doing	One Way I Can Improve
Rate yourself on eating a diet low in sugar. ☐ **Excellent:** I eat very few foods that contain a lot of added sugar. ☐ **Good:** I eat some foods that contain a lot of added sugar. ☐ **Fair:** Every day, some of the foods I eat contain added sugar. ☐ **Poor:** Every day, many of the foods I eat contain added sugar.	

(continued)

Assessing My Eating Habits (continued)

▶ Guideline 5

Eat less salt.

Most people eat too much salt. Snack foods such as chips, french fries, crackers, and processed, prepackaged and frozen meals contain high amounts of salt.

How I'm Doing	One Way I Can Improve
Rate yourself on eating a diet low in salt. ☐ **Excellent:** I rarely salt my foods or eat foods high in salt. ☐ **Good:** I only occasionally salt my foods or eat foods high in salt. ☐ **Fair:** I sometimes salt my foods and eat some foods high in salt. ☐ **Poor:** I usually salt my foods and eat a lot of foods high in salt.	

▶ Guideline 6

Vary your protein routine.

Choose a variety of different sources of protein, such as seafood, eggs, beans, peas and nuts in addition to meats such as chicken, pork or beef to be sure you get all the nutrients you need.

How I'm Doing	One Way I Can Improve
Rate yourself on varying your protein routine. ☐ **Excellent:** I eat 5 to 7 ounces of protein each day from a wide variety of different sources, including fish. ☐ **Good:** I eat 5 to 7 ounces of protein from a few different sources. ☐ **Fair:** I eat 5 to 7 ounces of protein from just one kind of meat. ☐ **Poor:** I rarely eat protein.	

> **Self-Check**
> ☐ I rated how I'm doing on all 6 guidelines.
> ☐ I listed 1 specific way I can improve for each guideline.

Food Detective

Directions: Jamie is a seventh grader who wants to eat healthy. Look at what Jamie ate today. Be a food detective by using some of the Guidelines for Healthy Eating to assess Jamie's choices and recommend changes that will help Jamie eat healthier.

What Jamie Ate Today

Breakfast
2 cups of shredded wheat cereal
1 cup of low-fat milk
1 cup of orange juice

Lunch
Double hamburger (two 3-ounce hamburger patties) with 2 slices of cheese on a sesame seed bun
1 tablespoon of mayonnaise
2-ounce bag of potato chips
16-ounce cola soft drink

Snack
16-ounce cola soft drink
2-ounce bag of tortilla chips
candy bar

Dinner
2 cups whole-wheat pasta with ½ cup of tomato sauce
1 cup of lettuce salad with 2 tablespoons of ranch dressing
1 piece of garlic bread
1 cup of low-fat frozen yogurt

Did Jamie meet the healthy eating guidelines?

▶ **Guideline 1: Make half your plate fruits and vegetables.**

What fruits and vegetables did Jamie eat today?	What are some changes Jamie could have made to include more fruits and vegetables?

Why is it important to eat plenty of fruits and vegetables?

(continued)

Food Detective (continued)

▶ **Guideline 2: Make at least half your grains whole grains.**

What grains did Jamie eat today?	Which of these were whole grains?

What are some changes Jamie could have made to include more whole grains?

▶ **Guideline 3: Eat less unhealthy fat.**

What foods did Jamie eat today that are high in fat?	What are some changes Jamie could have made to eat less unhealthy fat?

Why is it important to limit the amount of unhealthy fat you eat?

▶ **Guideline 4: Eat less added sugar.**

What foods did Jamie eat today that are high in sugar?	What are some changes Jamie could have made to eat less sugar?

Why is it important to limit the amount of sugar you eat?

(continued)

© ETR   HEALTH*Smart* Middle School

Food Detective (continued)

► **Guideline 5: Eat less salt.**

What salty foods did Jamie eat today?	What are some changes Jamie could have made to eat less salt?
Why is it important to limit the amount of salt you eat?	

► **Guideline 6: Vary your protein routine.**

What protein foods did Jamie eat today?	What are some choices Jamie could have made to vary the protein routine?
Why is it important to vary your protein routine?	

What advice do you have?

What advice would you give to Jamie about the benefits of eating in moderation?_____

_____

_____

_____

Make up a new menu for 1 meal that would help Jamie follow the guidelines for healthy eating and improve nutrition for the day: _____

_____

_____

_____

Self-Check
- ☐ I answered the questions about each guideline.
- ☐ I wrote advice about eating in moderation.
- ☐ I made up a more-nutritious menu for 1 meal.

Student Journal
Reading a Food Label

Journal entry

Take out the food label you brought from home and study it.

What information does it contain?

_____

_____

_____

What nutrients does it list?

_____

_____

_____

Food labels

How do you think the information on a food label could help you make healthier food choices?

_____

_____

_____

Healthy behavior

Eating the right number of servings from each food group every day, and eating less unhealthy fat, added sugar and salt.

Health terms

calorie

cholesterol

gram

high blood pressure

lean

milligram

processed foods

saturated fat

sodium

trans fat

What's a calorie?

- A calorie is _____.
- The number of calories you need depends on _____.
- Middle school students need between _____ and _____ calories a day.

Processed foods – Foods that have been changed so they will last longer, taste different or be faster to prepare. They usually come in a box or bag and may have added sugar, salt and unhealthy fat.

© ETR HEALTH*Smart* Middle School

Anatomy of a Food Label

2 Servings per Container and Serving Size

Serving sizes are given in common units, such as cups or pieces, followed by the metric amount, such as the number of grams. Serving sizes are based on the amount of food people typically eat, which makes them easy to compare to similar foods.

Servings per container is there because people often eat more than the listed serving size. This means they need to multiply the number of calories per serving by the number of servings they actually eat.

4 Total Fat

This section shows the total fat in grams, and then tells how much of that total amount comes from both saturated and trans fat. You want to limit how much you eat of these unhealthy forms of fat.

Nutrition Facts

8 servings per container

Serving size   **1 cup (55g)**

Amount per serving

Calories   230

	% Daily Value*
Total Fat 8g	**10%**
Saturated Fat 1g	**5%**
Trans Fat 0g	
Cholesterol 0mg	**0%**
Sodium 160mg	**7%**
Total Carbohydrate 37g	**13%**
Dietary Fiber 4g	**14%**
Total Sugars 12g	
Includes 10g Added Sugars	**20%**
Protein 3g	

Vitamin D 2mcg	10%
Calcium 260mg	20%
Iron 8mg	45%
Potassium 235mg	6%

* The % Daily Value (DV) tells you how much a nutrient in a serving of food contributes to a daily diet. 2,000 calories a day is used for general nutrition advice.

---

1 Calories

Calories provide a measure of how much energy you get from a serving of this food.

3 Carbohydrates

This section shows the total carbohydrates in grams, and then tells how much of that is from dietary fiber and how much is from sugars.

6 Added Sugars

The label also shows how much of the total sugar is from added sugars, rather than the sugar that occurs naturally in the food. Limiting added sugars is important for good health.

7 Sodium

You also want to limit how much sodium, or salt, you eat. Teens should average no more than 2,300 miligrams (mg) of sodium a day.

5 Vitamins and Minerals

The label shows how much the food contains of some important vitamins and minerals.

Label Detective

Directions: Compare the food labels you and your partner brought from home. Then answer the questions. Attach the labels to this sheet when you are done.

(1) What 2 foods are you comparing?   1. _____   and   2. _____

(2) What are the serving sizes?   Food label 1 _____   Food label 2 _____

(3) How many total servings per container?

Food label 1 _____   Food label 2 _____

(4) Which food has:

	Food label 1	Food label 2
fewer calories per serving?	☐	☐
less saturated fat?	☐	☐
less trans fat?	☐	☐
less sodium (salt)?	☐	☐
less added sugar?	☐	☐

(5) Which food would be the healthier choice? _____
Why? _____

_____

If you ate the whole container, would your answer change? Why?

_____

_____

(6) How can food labels help improve your eating habits? Give at least 2 examples.

_____

_____

_____

_____

_____

Self-Check
- ☐ We found and compared all the information from the 2 labels.
- ☐ We compared the nutrition values of the 2 foods and decided which is healthier.
- ☐ We explained how food labels can improve eating habits and gave 2 specific examples.

© ETR   HEALTH*Smart* Middle School

Lesson 5

Healthy behavior

Eating breakfast every day.

Health terms

barrier

calorie

fast

metabolism

protein

Student Journal
Eating Breakfast Every Day

Journal entry

List what you ate for breakfast this morning and describe how you are feeling right now. If you didn't eat breakfast, write your reasons and describe how you are feeling right now.

_____

_____

_____

_____

_____

> **Metabolism – How fast or slow your body burns calories.**

Benefits of eating a healthy breakfast

- ☐ Provides energy
- ☐ Helps reduce hunger
- ☐ Improves alertness
- ☐ Helps you concentrate better in school
- ☐ Improves memory
- ☐ Helps you get better grades and test scores
- ☐ Increases school attendance and decreases tardiness
- ☐ Leads to fewer discipline problems in school
- ☐ May help reduce obesity
- ☐ Leads to fewer visits to the school nurse

Check the 2 benefits that are most important to you.

(continued)

Student Journal
Eating Breakfast Every Day (continued)

Reason for not eating breakfast	How to overcome it

Healthy breakfast guidelines

A healthy breakfast should include:

Fruit — fresh, dried or 100% fruit juice

_____

_____

Whole-grain foods — whole-grain hot and cold cereals, whole-grain bread, pancakes made with whole-grain flour

_____

_____

A source of protein — milk or other dairy products, meat, eggs, beans

_____

_____

HEALTHSmart Middle School

© ETR

Breakfast: Benefits & Barriers

Directions: Think about what you learned today about eating breakfast, then answer the questions.

1 Which 2 benefits of eating breakfast are most important to you and why?

1. _____

_____

2. _____

_____

2 List at least 2 examples of foods you could eat for breakfast that meet each Healthy Breakfast Guideline.

A healthy breakfast should include:	Foods that meet this guideline	
fruit		
whole-grain foods		
a source of protein		

3 Name 2 potential barriers to eating breakfast that apply to you, and suggest at least 1 good way to overcome each of them.

Barrier 1: _____   Barrier 2: _____

_____   _____

How to overcome it: _____   How to overcome it: _____

_____   _____

4 How could you improve your own breakfast habits? Explain at least 1 thing you will do. Be specific.

_____

_____

_____

_____

_____

_____

Self-Check
☐ I listed 2 benefits of eating breakfast and explained why each is important to me.
☐ I listed at least 2 examples of foods that meet each Healthy Breakfast Guideline.
☐ I named 2 barriers to eating breakfast and explained how to overcome each one.
☐ I explained at least 1 way I will improve my breakfast habits.

Healthy behavior

Eating healthy snacks.

Health terms

characteristic

commercial

processed foods

snack

Student Journal
Healthy Snacking

Journal entry

List what you ate for snacks or between meals yesterday. Next to each item, write which food group it was from. Then put a + sign next to the snacks you think were healthy.

Snack	Food Group	Healthy?

Characteristics of a healthy snack

- Tasty
- Smaller in size than a meal
- Provides key nutrients
- Low in unhealthy fat
- Low in added sugar
- Low in salt

Speed write

You'll have 2 minutes to list as many healthy snacks as you can. Be sure they're snacks you would really eat.

_____

_____

_____

_____

_____

Healthy Snack Score

© ETR **HEALTH**Smart Middle School

Healthy Snacks

Directions: List 3 different healthy snack foods that you would really eat. Beside each snack food, explain which characteristics of a healthy snack it meets.

▶ Part 1

Healthy snack	Why it's healthy
1. _____	_____
	_____
2. _____	_____
	_____
3. _____	_____
	_____

▶ Part 2

From your lists in Part 1 choose the healthy snack that you and your partner like the best.

Prepare a 1-minute commercial that teens would like to convince your classmates to eat this snack on a regular basis. Make sure your commercial:

1. Would convince people your age.
2. Gives the name and a description of the food.
3. Explains why this snack is good to eat.
4. Explains why it's a healthy choice.
5. Explains why everyone should choose it as a snack food.
6. Lasts just 1 minute or less.

Fact
Snacking moderately throughout the day can help people control hunger and maintain a healthy weight.

You and your partner both need to be in the commercial. You can use pictures or props.

_____
_____
_____
_____
_____
_____

Self-Check
☐ We named 3 different snacks that meet the characteristics.
☐ We explained why each snack is healthy.
☐ Our commercial contains all 6 of the criteria.
☐ Our commercial appeals to teens.

© ETR HEALTH*Smart* Middle School

Healthy behavior

Eating healthy foods when dining out.

Health terms

au gratin

basted

beverage

broiled

grilled

hollandaise

intake

scalloped

Student Journal

Eating Healthy at Fast-Food Restaurants

Journal entry

List some of the snacks you've eaten since the last class.

_____

_____

_____

_____

Were they mainly healthy choices? Why or why not?

_____

_____

_____

My last fast-food meal

Describe or draw what you ate the last time you went to a fast-food restaurant. If you haven't eaten fast food, describe or draw a typical meal you imagine someone your age would order at one of these restaurants.

(continued)

© ETR **HEALTH** *Smart* Middle School

Student Journal
Eating Healthy at
Fast-Food Restaurants *(continued)*

Our top 5 ways to eat healthy at restaurants

1. _____

_____

2. _____

_____

3. _____

_____

4. _____

_____

5. _____

_____

My new fast-food meal

Describe or draw the changes you would make to the fast-food meal you described or drew at the beginning of class to make it healthier.

Fast-Food Meals

> **Directions:** Estimate the amount of calories, fat and salt in each meal on the left-hand side of the page. When your teacher tells you to, estimate the amount of calories, fat and salt in each meal on the right-hand side of the page, and explain why each of these meals, including the drinks, is healthier.

Fast-Food Meals

1 Quarter-pound cheeseburger, large fries, 16 oz. chocolate milkshake

_____ calories   _____ g fat   _____ mg sodium

2 4 slices sausage and mushroom pizza, 16 oz. soda

_____ calories   _____ g fat   _____ mg sodium

3 2 pieces fried chicken (breast and wing), buttermilk biscuit, mashed potatoes and gravy, corn on the cob, 16 oz. soda

_____ calories   _____ g fat   _____ mg sodium

4 Taco salad, 16 oz. soda

_____ calories   _____ g fat   _____ mg sodium

Recommended DAILY intake:*

Calories   1,800–2,400
Fat   No more than 50–80 g
Sodium   No more than 2,300 mg

*Calories are for a moderately active middle school student.

Healthier Fast-Food Meals

1 Hamburger, small fries, 8 oz. carton of 1% milk

_____ calories   _____ g fat   _____ mg sodium

This meal is healthier because:

_____

_____

2 3 slices vegetarian pizza, 16 oz. unsweetened iced tea

_____ calories   _____ g fat   _____ mg sodium

This meal is healthier because:

_____

_____

3 Broiled chicken sandwich, mashed potatoes and gravy, cole slaw, water

_____ calories   _____ g fat   _____ mg sodium

This meal is healthier because:

_____

_____

4 3 small tacos, 12 oz. apple juice

_____ calories   _____ g fat   _____ mg sodium

This meal is healthier because:

_____

_____

> **Self-Check**
> ☐ We guessed the amounts for each meal.
> ☐ We talked about how the foods are prepared.
> ☐ We explained which meals are healthier.

© ETR   HEALTH*Smart* Middle School

Healthy behavior

Preventing food-borne illnesses.

Health terms

bacteria

contaminated

expiration date

food-borne illness

germ

poultry

toxin

utensils

virus

Student Journal
Keeping Food Safe to Eat

Journal entry

Describe what you did to make your last fast-food meal healthier. If you haven't eaten in a fast-food restaurant since the last class, describe what you plan to do to make healthier choices next time you eat fast food.

_____

_____

_____

_____

_____

_____

Steps to take to keep food safe

Clean:

_____

_____

_____

Separate:

_____

_____

Chill:

_____

_____

Cook:

_____

_____

A Day in the Life of Dillon

Directions: Read the story. As you read, underline all of the things that might have put Dillon at risk for getting a food-borne illness. Then answer the questions.

Dillon woke up on Saturday morning to the smell of cooking—Dad was making a surprise breakfast. Dillon's dad started making an omelet by mixing several eggs with some milk that had been in the refrigerator for a while. Then Dad cut up a raw chicken breast on a cutting board and began cooking it in a skillet. Dad used the same knife and cutting board to chop some onion and tomato, and put them into the skillet with the chicken. Then Dad poured the egg mixture into the skillet without checking to see how well the chicken was cooked.

While the omelet was cooking, Dillon's dad made a fruit salad by cutting up some grapes, strawberries and bananas using the same cutting board and knife that he used before. After the food was ready, Dillon and Dad sat down to a tasty breakfast.

After breakfast, Dillon went over to Alex's house to play some basketball. After their first game, they went into the house for a snack. Alex asked if Dillon wanted some leftover pizza that was sitting out on the kitchen counter in a pizza box. They both had a piece and then went back out to play more basketball.

Then Dillon went home to finish some homework and decided to eat some leftover soup for lunch. Dillon warmed the soup up in the microwave. There were some cold spots, but Dillon was anxious to get the homework done, so didn't bother heating the soup more before eating it.

That evening, Dillon's family decided to go out to eat. Dillon ordered a hamburger, a salad and a glass of milk. The cook at the restaurant had just gone to the bathroom, but forgot to wash his hands before making Dillon's hamburger. Before the server made Dillon's salad, she finished clearing two tables and cashed out two checks. Then she reached into a bag of lettuce, grabbed enough to fill a bowl, and added a few tomatoes and cucumbers without washing her hands first.

They all enjoyed their dinner out, but later that night Dillon started feeling really sick.

What are at least 3 ways that Dillon could have become sick with a food-borne illness?

1. _____

_____

_____

2. _____

_____

_____

3. _____

_____

_____

What are at least 2 things Dillon could have done to prevent getting a food-borne illness?

1. _____

_____

_____

2. _____

_____

_____

Self-Check
☐ I underlined in the story all of the ways Dillon could have gotten a food-borne illness and explained 3 of them.
☐ I explained at least 2 ways Dillon could have prevented getting a food-borne illness.

Lesson 9

Healthy behavior

Eating less unhealthy fat, added sugar and salt, and eating healthy snacks.

Health terms

advertising

celebrity

external

influence

internal

media

negative

positive

technique

Student Journal
What Influences My Food Choices?

Journal entry

Review Part 1 of your **Food Diary**. Then complete Part 2.

> **Influence** – **To change someone's thoughts, beliefs or behaviors.**

Influences on food choices

1. _____
   + _____
   − _____

2. _____
   + _____
   − _____

3. _____
   + _____
   − _____

4. _____
   + _____
   − _____

5. _____
   + _____
   − _____

Ways to resist negative influences

Influence	Things I could do
1.	
2.	
3.	

(continued)

Student Journal
What Influences My Food Choices? *(continued)*

Food advertising techniques

Appeal to feelings: _____

_____

Example: _____

Toys and games: _____

_____

Example: _____

Famous people: _____

_____

Example: _____

Everyone eats it: _____

_____

Example: _____

Easy and fast: _____

_____

Example: _____

Value: _____

_____

Example: _____

Taste: _____

_____

Example: _____

Health: _____

_____

Example: _____

Food Diary

Directions: Over the next 24 hours, complete this food diary. In the first column, write what you eat for each snack or meal and fill out the chart in Part 1. You will complete Parts 2, 3 and 4 in class.

▶ Part 1: Keep Track of What You Eat

What did you eat?	When did you eat?	Where did you eat? (home, friend's house, watching TV, etc.)	With whom did you eat?	What was your mood?	How hungry were you?	How healthy was the meal or snack?
					☐ not hungry ☐ hungry ☐ very hungry	☐ not healthy ☐ somewhat healthy ☐ healthy
					☐ not hungry ☐ hungry ☐ very hungry	☐ not healthy ☐ somewhat healthy ☐ healthy
					☐ not hungry ☐ hungry ☐ very hungry	☐ not healthy ☐ somewhat healthy ☐ healthy
					☐ not hungry ☐ hungry ☐ very hungry	☐ not healthy ☐ somewhat healthy ☐ healthy
					☐ not hungry ☐ hungry ☐ very hungry	☐ not healthy ☐ somewhat healthy ☐ healthy
					☐ not hungry ☐ hungry ☐ very hungry	☐ not healthy ☐ somewhat healthy ☐ healthy
					☐ not hungry ☐ hungry ☐ very hungry	☐ not healthy ☐ somewhat healthy ☐ healthy
					☐ not hungry ☐ hungry ☐ very hungry	☐ not healthy ☐ somewhat healthy ☐ healthy

(continued)

Food Diary (continued)

▶ Part 2: Assess Your Patterns

How many meals/snacks did you eat:

____ at home	____ with your family	____ while you were watching TV
____ at school	____ alone	____ because of a certain mood
____ "on the go"	____ with a friend	____ when you weren't hungry

▶ Part 3: Analyze Influences

① When and where did you eat the healthiest? What was the biggest positive influence on your healthy choices?

_____

_____

_____

_____

② When and where did you eat the least healthy? What was the biggest negative influence on your less-healthy choices?

_____

_____

_____

_____

③ If you did eat a meal or snack when you weren't hungry, what influenced you to eat it?

_____

_____

_____

④ What did you learn about the influences on your eating habits and food choices?

_____

_____

_____

_____

(continued)

© ETR **HEALTH**Smart Middle School

Food Diary (continued)

▶ Part 4: What Will You Do?

(1) Based on what you learned, name at least 1 thing you personally plan to do to make healthier food choices in the future.

_____

_____

_____

_____

_____

(2) Describe 1 way you could counter or resist a negative influence on your food choices.

_____

_____

_____

_____

_____

_____

Self-Check
☐ I filled out the chart in Part 1 completely.

☐ I assessed my patterns in Part 2.

☐ I analyzed the influences on my choices in Part 3.

☐ I explained 1 way I can eat healthier and how I can counter a negative influence in Part 4.

Healthy behavior

Eating less unhealthy fat, added sugar and salt; eating healthy snacks; and eating healthy when dining out.

Health terms

alternative

body language

peers

pressure line

resisting pressure

roleplay

Student Journal
Resisting Pressure to Eat Less-Healthy Foods

Journal entry

Do you think it's easy or hard to counter or resist negative influences? Why?

_____

_____

_____

_____

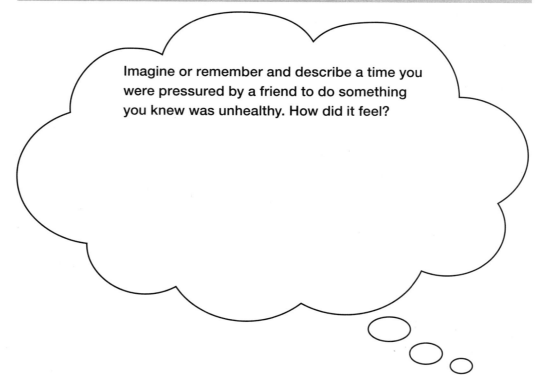

Imagine or remember and describe a time you were pressured by a friend to do something you knew was unhealthy. How did it feel?

Peer influences

What are some ways friends might influence a person to eat less-nutritious foods?

_____

_____

_____

(continued)

Student Journal
Resisting Pressure to
Eat Less-Healthy Foods *(continued)*

Pressure lines

What are some things friends might say to pressure you into eating less-nutritious foods?

1. _____
   _____
   _____
   _____

2. _____
   _____
   _____
   _____

3. _____
   _____
   _____
   _____

Saying NO to pressure

- Say NO.
- Use body language and actions that support the NO message.
- Suggest an alternative.
- Repeat.

Be sure your words and actions are real for the situation, are believable, and would work with the people you know.

My additional notes

_____
_____
_____
_____
_____

Resisting Food Pressures

> **Directions:** Read your group's assigned Food Pressure Scenario, and the pressure line Person A says. Then work on your own to write a response for Person B that says NO to the pressure and includes a realistic alternative Person B can suggest. Think about what body language you will use to reinforce the NO in Person B's response.

Food Pressure Scenarios

☐ **1. Which Lunch Line?**

Two friends go to the cafeteria for their lunch period. Person B heads toward the school lunch line. Person A starts going toward the a la carte line.

Pressure Line—Person A:

School lunches are boring. I'm going to get fries and pizza. Do you want to split them with me?

Response—Person B: _____
(write your name here)

☐ **2. Hungry After School**

Person B is at person A's house after school. They both feel hungry.

Pressure Line—Person A:

I'm starving. Do you want chips or cookies with your soda?

Response—Person B: _____
(write your name here)

(continued)

Resisting Food Pressures

(continued)

☐ **3. Have a Cheeseburger**

Person A and Person B are at a fast-food restaurant. Person A orders a double cheeseburger, large fries and a coke.

Pressure Line—Person A:

Do you want me to order you the same thing?

Response—Person B: _____

(write your name here)

☐ **4. Fast-Food Lunch Choice**

Person B packed a lunch from home, but Person A wants to go out for lunch at a new fast-food restaurant.

Pressure Line—Person A:

Let's try that new place. I heard they have great nachos.

Response—Person B: _____

(write your name here)

☐ **5. Study Snacks**

Two friends are meeting to study for a big test. Person A shows up at Person B's house with a big bag of candy and some energy drinks.

Pressure Line—Person A:

This will give us lots of energy to stay up and study.

Response—Person B: _____

(write your name here)

Self-Check

☐ I wrote a response for Person B that says NO and fits the situation.

☐ I wrote a healthy alternative for Person B to suggest.

☐ I included at least 1 action to reinforce the NO.

☐ I wrote a response to the pressure line that is real and believable and would work with the people I know.

Observer Feedback Form

> **Directions:** Practice your roleplay with your group. Take turns playing Person A, Person B and Observer.

Observer Feedback by: _____
(Write your name here)

I watched a roleplay by _____
(Name of student playing Person A)

and _____ .
(Name of student playing Person B)

As you watch the roleplay, check off the ways to say NO that Person B uses.

☐ Said NO.

Notes: _____

_____

_____

☐ Used a firm tone of voice.

Notes: _____

_____

_____

☐ Body language supported the NO.

Notes: _____

_____

_____

☐ Suggested an alternative.

Notes: _____

_____

_____

☐ Words and actions were real for the situation.

Notes: _____

_____

_____

☐ Would work with people you know.

Notes: _____

_____

_____

Lesson 11

Healthy behavior

Analyze influences on body image to support eating healthy and being physically active.

Health terms

appearance

attractive

average

body image

culture

genes

media

negative body image

positive body image

Student Journal
Body Image Basics

Journal entry

On a separate piece of paper, write a few sentences or draw a picture that expresses how you feel about your body. This will be private. You won't have to share it.

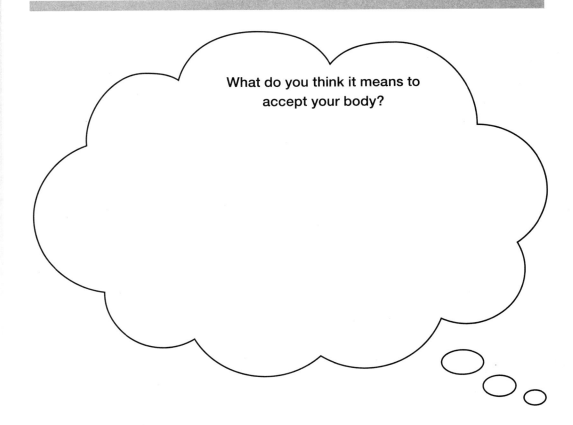

What do you think it means to accept your body?

Body image – The view you have of your body—size, weight, shape, looks—and your feelings about it.

Positive body image – Having a view of your body that's healthy and realistic, appreciating and valuing your unique body, and understanding that it's the whole person that's important—not just how you look.

(continued)

Influences on body image

(Put a star by the one you are assigned.)

Culture	**+**	**−**

Family	**+**	**−**

Friends	**+**	**−**

Media	**+**	**−**

Body Image Facts

▶ Did You Know That...

Media messages influence how our culture defines what it means to be attractive. The media influence how people view their bodies and how they feel about themselves.

Fact

Ads are made to convince you to buy or support a product or service.

Fact

Advertisers create their messages based on what they think you will want to see and what they think will get you to buy their product.

Fact

Over 47% of high school students say they are trying to lose weight.

Fact

Nearly 1 out of every 4 TV ads sends some sort of "attractiveness message" that tells viewers what is or isn't attractive. This means the average teen sees over 5,260 "attractiveness messages" a year.

Fact

Less than 16% of high school students are actually overweight. But twice that number think they are.

Fact

Over 20% of teens watch over 3 hours of television each day; 43% play video or computer games or spend time online for something besides schoolwork 3 or more hours a day.

Fact

About 3/4 of the fitness articles in teen magazines state that the main reason to exercise is to become more attractive. About half say that losing weight or burning calories is the reason to be physically active.

Sources: National Eating Disorders Association, www.nationaleatingdisorders.org; CDC, Youth Risk Behavior Survey, www.cdc.gov/healthyyouth/yrbs; Mirror Mirror Eating Disorder Help, www.mirror-mirror.org/media-influence-on-body-image.htm

Steps to a Positive Body Image

Directions: Read these steps. Add any steps of your own that you want to. Then circle the 2 or 3 that will work for you.

There's no simple way to turn negative body image thoughts and actions into positive ones. Here are some ideas. You may be able to add others.

Surround yourself with positive people who like you for who you are and not just how you look.

Be realistic. Bodies come in all shapes and sizes.

Become a critic of media messages about bodies.

Eat healthy. Include lots of fresh vegetables and fruits, whole grains and water. Cut down on unhealthy fats and sweets.

Be nice to yourself. Relax. Exercise. Take a nap. Hang out with friends. Make time for you.

Add your own ideas:

_____
_____
_____
_____
_____

Develop a list of all the things you like about yourself. Review it often.

Wear comfortable clothes that make you feel good about your body.

Appreciate the things your body can do. Run. Dance. Breathe. Laugh. Be active every day.

Notice when you feel bad about your body. See if you can shift to more positive thoughts.

Instead of worrying about how you look, help others who are less fortunate than you. Acts of kindness will make you feel good about yourself.

Circle 2 or 3 steps you intend to use to develop or keep having a positive body image.

Body Image & Me

Directions: Think about what you've learned today, then answer the questions.

+

(1) **What does it mean to have a positive body image?**

_____

_____

_____

_____

–

What does it mean to have a negative body image?

_____

_____

_____

_____

(2) **Why do you think it's important to have a positive body image?**

(3) **Describe at least 3 things that can influence a person's body image:**

1. _____

_____

_____

2. _____

_____

_____

3. _____

_____

_____

Which of these things do you think has the greatest influence on you? How does it influence you? Be specific and give at least 1 example.

_____

_____

_____

_____

_____

_____

_____

_____

(continued)

© ETR   **HEALTH**Smart Middle School

Body Image & Me (continued)

④ Explain at least 2 steps a person can take to develop or keep up a positive body image.

1.

2.

⑤ Explain when you will use these steps and how they will help you.

_____

_____

_____

_____

_____

_____

_____

_____

Self-Check
- ☐ I defined positive body image and explained why it's important.
- ☐ I named 3 influences on body image.
- ☐ I explained how at least 1 of these influences affects me personally.
- ☐ I named at least 2 steps a person can take to develop or keep up a positive body image.
- ☐ I explained when I will use these steps and how they will help me.

© ETR **HEALTH**Smart Middle School

© ETR HEALTHSmart Middle School

Lesson 12

Healthy behavior

Preventing health problems that result from diet fads or trends.

Health terms

addictive

body mass index (BMI)

dehydrated

dehydration

diarrhea

dieting

fad diet

metabolic rate

metabolism

puberty

supplement

weight management

Student Journal
Dieting Dangers & Healthy Ways to Manage Weight

Journal entry

What's one way that having a positive body image can help you stay healthy?

_____

_____

_____

_____

10 Things to know about dieting

What did you learn about the dangers of dieting from the reading? _____

_____

_____

What did you learn about healthy ways to lose weight? _____

_____

_____

_____

Things People Do to Try to Lose Weight	Potential Problems
Skipping meals	
Not eating certain foods or eating only one type of food	
Counting calories	

(continued)

Things People Do to Try to Lose Weight	Potential Problems
Exercising	
Following a popular or fad diet	
Using weight-loss drugs or supplements	

Healthy ways to manage weight

1. Check with a doctor or registered dietitian.

   _____

   _____

2. Eat a healthy breakfast.

   _____

   _____

3. Eat healthy snacks.

   _____

   _____

4. Be physically active.

   _____

   _____

5. Balance what you eat with physical activity.

   _____

   _____

10 Things to Know About Dieting

(1) **Losing weight isn't always healthy.** In fact, it's more dangerous to be 30% underweight than 30% overweight.

(2) **People's genes affect their weight.** Certain body shapes run in families. Dieting can't change this.

(3) **Dieting rarely works.** About 95% of people who lose weight by dieting gain back the weight they lost in 4 to 5 years. Over time, many people who've dieted end up weighing more than when they started.

(4) **There's only one sure way to lose weight.** You need to reduce the number of calories you eat, or increase the number of calories you burn off through physical activity. Most experts recommend doing both.

(5) **Dieting can mean people miss out on key nutrients.** For example, dieters often don't get enough calcium. Lack of nutrients is why very low-calorie diets are dangerous.

(6) **Some people who diet lose and gain weight back over and over.** This is called "yo-yo" dieting. Yo-yo dieting can change the way your body uses food, so you may end up gaining instead of losing weight when you yo-yo diet.

(7) **Dieting can lower the rate at which your body burns calories when you're resting or sitting still.** This means that after you stop dieting, your body uses the energy from food more slowly. So it's easier for you to gain weight on fewer calories.

(8) **Many diet trends tend to focus on reducing or increasing certain foods or nutrients.** Some focus on when and how much you eat. Some of these recommendations may be OK and help people lose weight or change their bodies. But it can be difficult for many people to stay on these fad diets for long periods of time, and eventually they gain the weight back.

(9) **Teens can gain anywhere from 20 to 50 pounds during a year of puberty.** This is natural. Some teens get taller first. Others get heavier first. Teens need to be patient. In time, the body will balance itself out.

(10) **To lose weight safely and keep it off, many experts say you should set a goal of a pound a week.** You can do this by eating 500 fewer calories per day, increasing your physical activity so you burn off 500 calories a day, or using a combination of eating and exercise (3,500 calories = 1 pound).

Weight a Minute: Advice from a Friend

Directions: Read each letter. Write an answer based on what you've learned about dieting and healthy weight management. Be sure to explain any dangers or potential problems with the strategies mentioned in the letters and offer advice on healthy ways to manage weight to each letter writer.

Dear Friend,

One of my friends went on a liquid diet she bought at the grocery store. She got only about 500 calories a day from the drinks. She lost weight, but she gained it all back when she quit drinking the diet stuff. Now she is thinking about going back on the liquid diet. She asked me for advice. How can I convince her that this kind of dieting is dangerous?

Concerned and Confused

(1) Dear Concerned and Confused,

_____
_____
_____
_____
_____
_____
_____
_____
_____
_____
_____

Dear Friend,

My best friend never eats in the morning and thinks it will be easy lose weight by skipping breakfast. My friend says it's just extra food the body doesn't need. I don't think what my friend is doing is healthy. What do you think?

Believes in Breakfast

(2) Dear Believes in Breakfast,

_____
_____
_____
_____
_____
_____
_____

(continued)

© ETR **HEALTH***Smart* Middle School

Weight a Minute: Advice from a Friend

(continued)

Dear Friend,

My brother is always listening to other people's ideas about "easy" ways to lose weight. He doesn't think that what he eats or how active he is matters. What can I recommend as healthy ways to manage his weight?

    Curious Sibling

(3) Dear Curious Sibling,

_____
_____
_____
_____
_____
_____
_____
_____

Dear Friend,

I saw an ad for this weight-loss pill online. It sounds great. The people on the website talked about how much weight they lost and how fast it was. Is there any reason I shouldn't try it? It's expensive, but they'll give you a 2-week supply free if you order it.

    Online for Weight Loss

(4) Dear Online for Weight Loss,

_____
_____
_____
_____
_____
_____
_____
_____

Fact

The best way to lose or maintain weight is to eat a varied, healthy diet and get regular physical activity.

Self-Check

☐ I identified the dangers of the diet strategies in the letters.

☐ I included healthy ways to manage weight in my responses.

☐ I explained how eating and exercise habits affect body weight in my response to letter 3.

☐ I described the dangers of using weight-loss pills in my response to letter 4.

Eating Disorders

Healthy behavior

Getting help for disordered eating or unhealthy physical activity patterns.

Health terms

anemia

anorexia nervosa

binge eating

bulimia nervosa

compulsive

consequence

constipation

disordered eating

diuretic

eating disorder

esophagus

excessive

heart rate

intense

irrational

lanugo

laxative

misperception

purge

self-starvation

symptom

Journal entry

Complete this sentence: If I ever needed to lose weight, I would take these 3 healthy steps:

1. _____

_____

_____

2. _____

_____

_____

3. _____

_____

_____

> **Disordered eating** – A range of unhealthy eating behaviors that may lead to development of an eating disorder.

Signs of disordered eating

Thoughts & Feelings	Behaviors
• Thinking about weight, food, dieting or exercising all the time	• Avoiding certain foods or food groups
• Basing self-worth and self-esteem only on body shape or weight	• Having set rituals or strict rules around eating and/or exercise
• Feeling worried or anxious about certain foods or food groups	• Skipping meals or avoiding social eating
• Feeling guilty or ashamed about eating	• Obsessive calorie counting or exercising
• Feeling out of control around food	• Eating compulsively
	• Using exercise, fasting or purging to "make up for eating bad foods"

(continued)

© ETR **HEALTH**Smart Middle School

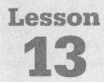

Lesson 13

Student Journal
Eating Disorders (continued)

How to help a friend

Things to do:

Express concern:

_____

_____

Listen:

_____

_____

Be supportive:

_____

_____

Encourage your friend to get help from professionals:

_____

_____

Things to avoid:

Don't try to change your friend's eating:

_____

_____

Don't take part in conversations about food, body size, calories or weight:

_____

_____

Don't give advice:

_____

_____

Where to get help

Who are some adults you could go to for help with disordered eating?

1. _____

2. _____

3. _____

© ETR   HEALTH*Smart* Middle School

Eating Disorders

Eating disorders are serious illnesses. People of any age can have an eating disorder, but they usually start when a person is a teen. They are more common in girls, but boys can also develop them. Eating disorders almost always require help from medical and mental health professionals.

There are two main types of eating disorders that teens should know about.

▶ Anorexia Nervosa

What Is Anorexia?

Anorexia is an extreme fear of body fat and gaining weight that leads to people starving themselves. It goes far beyond normal concerns about eating or being thin. The fear of fat is irrational—it's not based on facts or reason. People with anorexia are so afraid of being "fat" that they starve themselves and lose a large amount of weight. Even though they are so underweight that they are hurting their bodies, they continue to want to lose weight.

Symptoms of Anorexia

People with anorexia:

- Avoid food and meals.
- Eat just a few foods in very small amounts.
- Weigh their food and/or count the calories in everything they eat or drink.
- Have a very distorted body image—they see themselves as "fat," even when they are very thin.
- May exercise too much as a way to lose even more weight.
- Are usually very thin and underweight.

Consequences

Anorexia causes many changes in the body and can result in serious health problems:

- Menstrual periods may stop.
- Heart rate slows down and blood pressure becomes very low. This increases the chances of heart failure.
- Hair and nails become brittle.
- Skin dries out and turns yellow.
- Eating so little means the body doesn't get the nutrients it needs. Bones become brittle due to loss of calcium. Anemia, or lack of iron in the blood, makes it hard for the blood to deliver enough oxygen to the body.
- Joints may swell, and the body loses muscle.
- The body forgets how to digest food. This can lead to constipation and pain in the abdomen.
- A covering of soft hair, called lanugo, grows on the body to help keep it warm.

(continued)

Eating Disorders (continued)

▶ Bulimia Nervosa

What Is Bulimia?

In bulimia, a person's concerns about gaining weight lead to bingeing and purging. Bingeing is eating a very large amount of food at one time. Purging is trying to get rid of that food by vomiting, or by using laxatives (drugs or other substances that cause bowel movements) or diuretics (drugs that get rid of excess water in the body). Almost everyone overeats once in a while, but people with bulimia do this often.

Symptoms of Bulimia

People with bulimia:

■ Feel out of control during a binge.

■ Feel guilty after a binge.

■ May spend a lot of time alone so that they can binge and purge in secret.

■ May also exercise to excess to get rid of calories eaten during a binge.

■ Often are normal weight or only slightly overweight.

Consequences

Bulimia can also cause serious health problems:

■ Acid from vomit wears down tooth enamel.

■ The stomach and esophagus (the tube that takes food from the mouth to the stomach) become damaged by the frequent vomiting.

■ Glands in the cheek enlarge. This makes the cheeks look swollen.

■ Loss of water due to purging can cause dehydration and damage the kidneys.

■ Loss of minerals such as potassium can lead to heart failure.

*Another eating disorder called **binge-eating disorder is similar to bulimia. But the person doesn't purge or overexercise to make up for the food eaten during a binge.***

Disordered Eating Scenarios

> **Directions:** Read the scenario assigned to your group. Describe the symptoms of disordered eating that you see in the scenario and explain how the person's behaviors are affecting their nutrition. Then write what you would say if the person in the story was your friend to encourage them to get help.

1. Anjoli's Story

Anjoli's friends tell her she's very thin, but she wants to be thinner. Anjoli spends a lot of time talking about how fat she is, especially in her stomach and thighs. She constantly counts calories and fat grams in food. At lunch, she often doesn't eat at all. When she does, she cuts her food up into really small pieces. By the time the bell rings, she has eaten only a small amount.

What signs of disordered eating is Anjoli showing? _____

_____

How are Anjoli's eating patterns affecting nutrition? _____

_____

If Anjoli was your friend, what would you say and do? _____

_____

2. Paul's Story

Paul has a secret weight loss plan. He loves to eat—especially sweet foods like ice cream, candy, cookies and cakes, but he doesn't want to gain weight. He sneaks food into his room and eats until he can't eat anymore. He feels ashamed, but he can't seem to stop. He then goes into the bathroom and makes himself vomit. He has bad breath or smells like mouthwash or mints all the time.

What signs of disordered eating is Paul showing? _____

_____

How are Paul's eating patterns affecting nutrition? _____

_____

If Paul was your friend, what would you say and do? _____

_____

(continued)

© ETR **HEALTH**Smart Middle School

Disordered Eating Scenarios

(continued)

3. D.J.'s Story

D.J. takes only tiny portions when eating and skips meals on a regular basis. Sometimes D.J. chews a mouthful of food and then spits it out before swallowing it. Most of the time, D.J. makes excuses not to eat, claiming to not be hungry, be feeling sick, or have already eaten.

What signs of disordered eating is D.J. showing? _____

_____

How are D.J.'s eating patterns affecting nutrition? _____

_____

If D.J. was your friend, what would you say and do? _____

_____

4. Cara's Story

Cara was scared that she was gaining weight and not getting any taller. She read that if she started taking laxatives, she could lose weight quickly. She started out taking 1 or 2 a day, but now she takes 10. Since she's been taking them, she seems stressed out and depressed.

What signs of disordered eating is Cara showing? _____

_____

How are Cara's eating patterns affecting nutrition? _____

_____

If Cara was your friend, what would you say and do? _____

_____

5. Regi's Story

Regi began exercising to get fit and lose some weight. Regi's doctor and P.E. teacher helped Regi start an exercise program. But now Regi is using exercise as a way to burn calories after eating too much. Regi is exercising before school for an hour, then lifting weights for an hour after school, and then running for another hour after dinner. Regi has lost weight and isn't looking very healthy, but still wants to exercise harder.

What signs of disordered eating is Regi showing? _____

_____

How are Regi's eating patterns affecting nutrition? _____

_____

_____

If Regi was your friend, what would you say and do? _____

_____

_____

Self-Check

☐ We identified all of the symptoms of disordered eating in our scenario.

☐ We described how the disordered eating affects proper nutrition.

☐ We explained what we would say and do to help the person in the story.

Student Journal
Assessing My Physical Activity

Healthy behavior

Engaging in the recommended amounts and types of physical activity every day.

Health terms

aerobic

cardiorespiratory

endurance

fitness

intensity

moderate

physical activity

physical fitness

strengthen

vigorous

Journal entry

Think about what you did this past week. Write down as many ways you were physically active, or moved your body in ways that required energy, as you can remember. Put a star by any activities that made your heart beat faster than it usually does.

_____

_____

_____

_____

_____

_____

How do you feel when you are physically active and move your body?

Fitness – Your body's ability to function at its best and meet the demands of life.

(continued)

© ETR **HEALTH** *Smart* Middle School

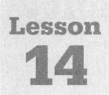

Lesson 14

Student Journal
Assessing My Physical Activity *(continued)*

Guidelines for physical activity

1. Be physically active for at least 60 minutes each day.

    aerobic = _____

    _____

    moderate = _____

    _____

2. Include vigorous-intensity aerobic activity on at least 3 days per week.

    vigorous = _____

    _____

    _____

3. Do muscle-strengthening activities on at least 3 days per week.

    _____

    _____

    _____

    _____

4. Do bone-strengthening activities on at least 3 days per week.

    _____

    _____

    _____

    _____

Ways I could add moderate or vigorous activity to my day

Assessing My Physical Activity

Directions: Read each guideline, rate yourself and list 1 realistic and specific way you could improve your activity habits to meet the guideline.

▶ Guideline 1

Be physically active for at least 60 minutes each day. Most of this should be moderate- to vigorous-intensity aerobic activity.

How I'm Doing	One Way I Can Improve
Rate yourself on your daily physical activity. ☐ **Excellent:** I spend 60 minutes each day doing things that count as physical activity. ☐ **Good:** I spend 30 to 60 minutes each day doing things that count as physical activity. ☐ **Fair:** I spend under 30 minutes each day doing things that count as physical activity. ☐ **Poor:** I am not physically active on most days.	

▶ Guideline 2

Include vigorous-intesity aerobic activities on at least 3 days per week.

How I'm Doing	One Way I Can Improve
Rate yourself on your vigorous aerobic activity level. ☐ **Excellent:** I do vigorous aerobic activity on 3 or more days per week. ☐ **Good:** I do vigorous aerobic activity on 2 days per week. ☐ **Fair:** I do vigorous aerobic activity on 1 day per week. ☐ **Poor:** I rarely do vigorous aerobic activity.	

(continued)

© ETR **HEALTH**Smart Middle School

Assessing My Physical Activity

(continued)

▶ Guideline 3

Do muscle-strengthening activities on at least 3 days per week.

How I'm Doing	One Way I Can Improve
Rate yourself on your muscle-strengthening activities. ☐ **Excellent:** I do muscle-strengthening activities on at least 3 days per week. ☐ **Good:** I do muscle-strengthening activities on 2 days per week. ☐ **Fair:** I do muscle-strengthening activities on 1 day per week. ☐ **Poor:** I rarely or never do muscle-strengthening activities	

▶ Guideline 4

Do bone-strengthening activities on at least 3 days per week.

How I'm Doing	One Way I Can Improve
Rate yourself on your bone-strengthening activities. ☐ **Excellent:** I do bone-strengthening activities on at least 3 days per week. ☐ **Good:** I do bone-strengthening activities on 2 days per week. ☐ **Fair:** I do bone-strengthening activities on 1 day per week. ☐ **Poor:** I do rarely or never do bone-strengthening activities.	

Self-Check
☐ I rated how I'm doing on all 4 guidelines.
☐ I listed 1 specific way I can improve for each guideline.

Activity Detective

Directions: Morgan is an eighth grader who wants to be physically fit. Look at Morgan's activity for the week. Be an activity detective by using the Guidelines for Physical Activity to assess Morgan's choices and recommend changes that will help Morgan get the right amount and types of physical activity.

▶ Morgan's Activity Log

Monday	Tuesday	Wednesday	Thursday
▪ walked to school (15 minutes) ▪ played basketball during lunch (20 minutes) ▪ walked home from school (15 minutes)	▪ walked to school (15 minutes) ▪ walked home from school (15 minutes)	▪ push-ups and sit-ups in the morning (5 minutes) ▪ walked to school (15 minutes) ▪ walked home from school (15 minutes)	▪ walked to school (15 minutes) ▪ walked home from school (15 minutes) ▪ bike ride with a friend (30 minutes)

Friday	Saturday	Sunday
▪ walked to school (15 minutes) ▪ walked home from school (15 minutes)	▪ soccer practice: push-ups and other exercises (20 minutes), running/ playing (60 minutes)	▪ walked to the park and home again (10 minutes each way)

Did Morgan meet the physical activity guidelines?

Guideline 1: Be physically active for at least 60 minutes each day. Most of this should be either moderate- or vigorous-intensity aerobic activity.

On which days was Morgan active for 60 minutes?	Which of Morgan's activities were moderate or vigorous?
☐ Monday ☐ Friday ☐ Tuesday ☐ Saturday ☐ Wednesday ☐ Sunday ☐ Thursday	

What are at least 3 ways Morgan could add more daily activity during the week?

1. _____

2. _____

3. _____

(continued)

© ETR **HEALTH**Smart Middle School

Activity Detective (continued)

Guideline 2: Include vigorous-intensity aerobic activity on at least 3 days per week.

On which days did Morgan do vigorous-intensity activities?	Why is aerobic activity important?
☐ Monday ☐ Friday ☐ Tuesday ☐ Saturday ☐ Wednesday ☐ Sunday ☐ Thursday	
What are at least 3 ways Morgan could add more vigorous-intensity activity to the week? 1. _____ 2. _____ 3. _____	

Guideline 3: Do muscle-strengthening activities on at least 3 days per week.

On which days did Morgan do muscle-strengthening activities?	How do muscle-strengthening activities improve your physical fitness?
☐ Monday ☐ Friday ☐ Tuesday ☐ Saturday ☐ Wednesday ☐ Sunday ☐ Thursday	
What are at least 3 activities Morgan could add to strengthen muscles? 1. _____ 2. _____ 3. _____	

(continued)

Activity Detective *(continued)*

Guideline 4: Do bone-strengthening activities on at least 3 days per week.

On which days did Morgan do bone-strengthening activities?	How do bone-strengthening activities improve your physical fitness?
☐ Monday ☐ Friday ☐ Tuesday ☐ Saturday ☐ Wednesday ☐ Sunday ☐ Thursday	

What are at least 3 activities Morgan could add to strengthen bones?

1. _____

2. _____

3. _____

What advice do you have?

Suggest at least 4 things Morgan could do next week to follow the guidelines and get more physical activity, without having to do a lot of planning or using special equipment.

1. _____

2. _____

3. _____

4. _____

Self-Check

☐ I listed at least 3 ways to increase daily activity to meet Guideline 1.

☐ I listed at least 3 examples of activities for Guidelines 2, 3 and 4.

☐ I listed at least 2 ways Morgan could increase aerobic activity next week.

☐ I listed at least 2 ways Morgan could increase muscle- and bone-strengthening activities next week.

☐ I listed activities that can be done without planning or special equipment.

© ETR **HEALTH**Smart Middle School

© ETR   **HEALTH**Smart Middle School

Healthy behavior

Avoiding injury during physical activity.

Health terms

cancer

chronic disease

climate

cool down

core body temperature

diabetes

flexibility

heart disease

heatstroke

high blood pressure

hydrated

hypothermia

muscle tone

osteoporosis

range of motion

sedentary

stress

type 2 diabetes

warm up

Student Journal
Staying Safe While Getting Fit

Journal entry

Describe any changes you've made to help meet the physical activity guidelines. If you didn't do anything to help meet the guidelines, write something you could do.

Benefits of physical activity	
Physical	Mental/Emotional
	Social

(continued)

Student Journal
Staying Safe While Getting Fit (continued)

Guidelines for staying safe during physical activity

1. Wear the proper safety equipment for the activity.

   What are some activities you do that require safety gear?

   _____

   _____

2. Protect yourself from climate and weather.

   What can you do to stay safe in different weather or climates when you're being active?

   _____

   _____

3. Drink plenty of water before, during and after physical activity.

   What are some ways to be sure you drink enough water before, during and after being active?

   _____

   _____

   _____

4. Warm up before physical activity.

   What are some things you can do to warm up before being active?

   _____

   _____

   _____

5. Cool down after physical activity.

   What are some things you can do to cool down after being active?

   _____

   _____

   _____

Staying Safe During Physical Activity

Directions: Use what you've learned to answer the questions.

1 You have a friend who doesn't see the point of being physically active. You know there are many physical, mental/emotional and social benefits of being physically active. What would you say to share at least 3 of these benefits with your friend?

_____

_____

_____

2 You have another friend who never wants to wear safety gear during sports. You are worried this friend could get injured. What would you say to convince your friend that it's important to wear safety gear when participating in certain physical activities?

_____

_____

_____

3 What are 2 climate-related conditions that can affect physical activity? For each one, describe something you could do to stay safer in these conditions.

_____

_____

4 You have a friend who doesn't drink water before, during or after being physically active. What would you say to convince your friend this is important?

_____

_____

_____

5 Why is it important to warm up before and cool down after physical activity?

_____

_____

_____

Self-Check

☐ I listed at least 3 benefits of physical activity.
☐ I explained the importance of safety gear.
☐ I described how weather and climate affect safety during physical activity.
☐ I explained why it's important to drink water when active.
☐ I explained the importance of warm-up and cool-down.

Student Journal
My Healthy Eating & Physical Activity Goal

Healthy behavior

Following an eating or physical activity plan to stay healthy.

Health terms

barrier

goal setting

measurable

realistic

specific

Journal entry

If you were going to choose one healthy eating or physical activity behavior to work on over the next few weeks, what would it be and why?

_____

_____

_____

_____

_____

_____

Setting a goal

1. What is your healthy eating or physical activity goal? (Be sure it's specific, realistic and measurable.) _____

    _____

2. What will be the benefits of reaching your goal? _____

    _____

3. Why is this goal important to you? _____

    _____

4. What must you do to reach this goal? _____

    _____

5. How will you start? _____

    _____

6. Who can help? _____

    _____

7. What could get in the way? _____

    _____

8   How can you adjust your plan if you need to? _____

    _____

Sample Healthy Eating & Physical Activity Goals

Directions: Here are some possible specific, realistic and measurable goals around healthy eating and physical activity. Review your **Assessing My Eating Habits** and **Assessing My Physical Activity** sheets to select a goal to work on. You can also write your own goal, if you want.

☐ I will eat 3 servings of vegetables a day for the next 2 weeks.

☐ I will drink 8 glasses of water a day for the next 30 days.

☐ I will eat one healthy snack a day this week.

☐ Any time I eat bread, I will eat whole-grain bread instead of white bread.

☐ I will eat 2 servings of fruit a day for the next 2 weeks.

☐ I will walk for 30 minutes, 4 days a week for the next month.

☐ I will warm up and stretch every time before I play basketball.

☐ I will do yoga 3 times a week for 30 minutes for the next 2 weeks

☐ I will ride my bike for 30 minutes 3 times a week for the next 2 weeks.

☐ I will substitute water for soda every time I eat at a fast-food restaurant.

☐ I will bring a healthy lunch to school at least 3 times a week.

▶ My Own Goal

© ETR HEALTH*Smart* Middle School

Healthy Eating & Physical Activity—*Getting Started*

Directions: Answer the following questions.

(1) What is your healthy eating or physical activity goal?

Is your goal:

☐ specific (it says exactly what you will do)

☐ realistic (you can do it)

☐ measurable (you'll know when you've reached it)

(2) What will be at least 2 benefits of reaching your goal?

_____

_____

_____

_____

(3) Why is this goal important to you?

_____

_____

_____

_____

_____

(4) What must you do to reach this goal?

_____

_____

_____

_____

_____

(continued)

© ETR **HEALTH**Smart Middle School

Healthy Eating & Physical Activity—*Getting Started*

(continued)

⑤ How will you start?

_____

_____

_____

_____

⑥ Who can help?

_____

_____

_____

_____

⑦ What could get in the way of reaching your goal?

Barrier	How I could over come it

⑧ Who will be your goal partner to help support you in reaching your goal?

_____

my partner's name

Self-Check

☐ I wrote a specific, realistic and measurable goal.

☐ I identified at least 2 benefits related to my goal.

☐ I identified at least 1 barrier and specific ways to overcome it.

☐ I completed each step on my plan with specific information.

Tracking My Progress

Healthy behavior

Following an eating or physical activity plan to stay healthy.

Health terms

abilities

monitor

priorities

responsibilities

Journal entry

How are you feeling about working on your goal? What's worked well? What's been challenging?

_____

_____

_____

_____

Do you want to adjust your goal to make it more challenging or easier?

_____

_____

Keeping on track

1. How are you doing?

2. What are you doing well?

3. Do you need to change anything to stay on track?

4. Who can help?

My additional notes

_____

_____

_____

_____

_____

_____

Eating & Physical Activity: Sample Plans

Here are examples of how 2 students kept track of their progress.

▶ Lavelle's Goal

Lavelle set a goal to build up to exercising for 30 minutes 3 times a week.

Monday

What steps did you take today to meet your goal?
I played soccer after school and stayed in the game the entire time.

What problem or barrier got in the way?	What did you do to overcome it?
None. I had fun.	Didn't need to.

Who helped you with your goal?
My teammates got into the game too.

Tuesday

What steps did you take today to meet your goal?
I walked home from school.

What problem or barrier got in the way?	What did you do to overcome it?
I didn't really walk fast enough for it to count as exercise.	I tried to speed up a bit. But I also know I'll get some good exercise tomorrow when I meet my friends to play basketball after school.

Who helped you with your goal?
My brother walked home with me.

What I Learned This Week

Things I did well:
I got good exercise from soccer on 2 days. And I played basketball with friends on Wednesday.

Benefits I enjoyed this week:
I felt proud about meeting my goal. I had more energy.

Problems I had and how I solved them:
Sometimes I feel too busy to exercise. Walking home from school is good physical activity, but I need to walk faster for it to count as exercise. I can ask my brother if he'll help me push the pace.

How I will adjust my goal plan:
No adjustment needed yet. I'm doing well.

What I am going to do toward my goal this weekend:
I'm going to play basketball with my friends again on Saturday.

(continued)

Eating & Physical Activity: Sample Plans *(continued)*

▶ Thomas's Goal

Thomas set a goal to eat fruits and vegetables 5 times a day.

Monday

What steps did you take today to meet your goal?
I carried an apple and some carrots with me in my backpack. I ate them for snacks.

What problem or barrier got in the way?	What did you do to overcome it?
My friends eat a lot of chips and things. It's really tempting to forget the fruit and to join them.	I offered my friends some of the carrots.

Who helped you with your goal?
My mom bought extra fruit when she went to the store. She helped me cut up vegetables to take for snacks tomorrow.

Tuesday

What steps did you take today to meet your goal?
When my friends went to the store after school to buy chips, I bought an orange instead.

What problem or barrier got in the way?	What did you do to overcome it?
I really wanted to eat cereal instead of carrot sticks for a snack after school.	I chose the whole-grain cereal and had a small bowl, but I also ate a few carrots too.

Who helped you with your goal?
I was on my own today.

What I Learned This Week

Things I did well:
I ate a vegetable with lunch and dinner and had 2 snacks that were fruit or vegetables on 4 out of 7 days.

Benefits I enjoyed this week:
I'm proud of myself for doing something healthy. I chose healthier foods overall too—not just the extra vegetables.

Problems I had and how I solved them:
I got a little bored with carrots. I'm going to go to the store with my mom to see what other kinds of fruit or vegetables would be quick and easy to carry. I'm still tempted to eat less-healthy snack foods when I'm with my friends. I try to get them to make healthier choices sometimes.

How I will adjust my goal plan:
I'm going to make my goal to eat fruits and vegetables 4 times a day for the next week. After I can meet that goal for a week, I'll increase it to 5 times a day.

What I am going to do toward my goal this weekend:
I'm going to prepare a lot of celery, red peppers and carrot sticks to eat for snacks.

Tracking My Progress

Directions: Write your eating or physical activity goal below. Complete the questions for each day of the week. On Friday, answer the questions about what you learned this week.

My goal:

Monday

What steps did you take today to meet your goal? _____

_____

_____

What problem or barrier got in the way?	What did you do to overcome it?

Who helped you with your goal? _____

Tuesday

What steps did you take today to meet your goal? _____

_____

_____

What problem or barrier got in the way?	What did you do to overcome it?

Who helped you with your goal? _____

(continued)

Tracking My Progress

(continued)

Wednesday

What steps did you take today to meet your goal? _____

_____

_____

What problem or barrier got in the way?	What did you do to overcome it?

Who helped you with your goal? _____

_____

Thursday

What steps did you take today to meet your goal? _____

_____

_____

What problem or barrier got in the way?	What did you do to overcome it?

Who helped you with your goal? _____

_____

(continued)

Tracking My Progress

(continued)

Friday

What steps did you take today to meet your goal? _____

_____

_____

What problem or barrier got in the way?	What did you do to overcome it?

Who helped you with your goal? _____

_____

▶ What I Learned This Week

■ **Things I did well:** _____

_____

_____

■ **Benefits I enjoyed this week:** _____

_____

_____

■ **Problems I had and how I solved them:** _____

_____

_____

■ **How I will adjust my goal plan:** _____

_____

_____

■ **What I am going to do toward my goal this weekend:** _____

_____

_____

Health Terms Glossary

abilities—The things a person is able to do, particularly the things the person is good at.

addictive—Relating to or causing physical and mental dependence on a drug.

advertising—Calling attention to products for sale through print, video, radio or other forms of media.

advocacy—Taking planned action to have a positive effect on other people's behaviors or the environment.

aerobic—Active only in the presence of oxygen. Aerobic activities are ones that move large muscle groups and make the heart and lungs work harder.

alternative—Something done or chosen instead of something else.

analyze—To examine in detail.

anemia—Lack of iron in the blood.

anorexia nervosa—An eating disorder characterized by underweight, fear of gaining weight and a distorted body image. It usually occurs in young women, is often accompanied by amenorrhea (loss of menstrual periods), and may be life threatening.

appearance—How something or someone looks.

attractive—Having qualities that are admired or get attention.

au gratin—Cooked with a crust of crumbs and grated cheese.

average—Usual or normal.

bacteria—One-celled microscopic organisms found in living things, air, soil and water. Some are beneficial to humans, but some cause disease.

barrier—Something that blocks, hinders or gets in the way.

basted—Moistened with melted butter, drippings, etc., while being cooked.

beverage—Any liquid for drinking.

binge eating—Consuming a large amount of food in a short time.

body image—The way people view their bodies, including size, weight and how attractive they are, and how they believe others view their bodies.

body language—The gestures, facial expressions and other physical clues that go with and can reinforce a verbal message; what a person is saying nonverbally with their body.

body mass index (BMI)—A measure of healthy weight, overweight and obesity based on the number of kilograms per square meter. It can be calculated by: (1) multiplying weight in pounds by 704; (2) squaring height in inches; (3) dividing the result of step 1 by the result of step 2. For adults, a BMI under 25 is healthy; 25–29.9 is overweight; and 30 or above is obese. For children and youth, a BMI at or over the 95th percentile is considered overweight.

Health Terms Glossary

(continued)

broiled—Cooked on a grill or rack by a heat source from above.

bulimia nervosa—An eating disorder that involves repeated, secret bouts of binge eating followed by purging (vomiting, fasting, use of laxatives or diuretics) or vigorous exercise in order to prevent weight gain.

calorie—A unit for measuring the energy produced by food when it is metabolized in the body.

campaign—A series of planned actions, as for electing a candidate or achieving some other result.

cancer—A disease that occurs when the body's cells grow in an out-of-control way.

carbohydrate—A nutrient composed of carbon, hydrogen and oxygen that provides the body's preferred form of energy.

cardiorespiratory—Relating to or involving the heart and lungs.

celebrity—A famous person.

characteristic—Trait or quality.

cholesterol—A waxy fat made by the body and an essential part of cell membranes; high levels in the blood can lead to heart disease.

chronic disease—An illness that lasts a long time or recurs often; can be treated but not cured.

climate—The prevailing weather conditions of a place.

commercial—An audio or visual advertisement for a product.

complex carbohydrates—Starch, glycogen and dietary fiber.

compulsive—Feeling compelled or forced, with no sense of control.

consequence—The result or outcome of an action or event.

constipation—Abnormally delayed or infrequent bowel movements that are hardened and dry.

contaminated—Infected by germs, such as bacteria; made unfit for use.

cool down—To slow the level of physical activity gradually to allow the heart and breathing to return to normal levels, to let the muscles recover, and to avoid other problems that can occur if activity is stopped suddenly.

core body temperature—Temperature inside the body, as opposed to the temperature of the outer areas.

counteract—To act in opposition to or neutralize the effect of something.

Health Terms Glossary

culture—The beliefs, behaviors, arts and social structures that people in a society learn, share and pass on to future generations.

dehydrated—Lacking adequate fluid in the body.

dehydration—Loss of fluid in the body.

diabetes (diabetes mellitus)—A chronic metabolic disorder in which the body's ability to use carbohydrates is impaired, while use of fats and protein is enhanced. A risk factor for cardiovascular disease, diabetes is linked with obesity and high blood pressure. Type 1 requires a person to take insulin, while type 2 may be controlled by diet.

diarrhea—Abnormally frequent and watery bowel movements.

diet—The overall combination of food and drink a person consumes over time.

dietary fiber— See *fiber*.

dieting—A short-term way to lose weight.

disordered eating—A range of unhealthy eating behaviors that may lead to development of an eating disorder.

diuretic—A substance or drug that increases the body's elimination of fluids.

eating disorder—A psychological illness characterized by disturbances in eating behavior.

endurance—The ability of muscles to keep doing an activity.

esophagus—The tube that carries food from the mouth to the stomach.

excessive—To an extreme degree, much more than is needed.

expiration date—The date something ends; the date after which a product may begin to spoil.

external—Coming from the outside world.

fad diet—A way of eating that suddenly becomes popular for a period of time.

fast—To eat sparingly or go without food.

fat—A nutrient that is the body's second major source of energy and the preferred means of storing energy.

fiber—Plant food components, including plant cell walls, pectins, gums and brans, that the body cannot digest.

fitness—A combination of qualities that allow an individual to meet the physical demands of life.

flexibility—The ability of joints to move through a full range of motion.

Health Terms Glossary

(continued)

food-borne illness—Illness caused by food that has been spoiled by harmful bacteria, toxins, parasites, viruses or chemicals.

food group—A collection of foods that share similar nutritional properties or biological classifications. Nutrition guides recommend daily servings of each food group for a healthy diet.

fortified—Enriched with added nutrients.

fructose—The sugar in sweet fruits and honey.

genes—The structures that pass inherited characteristics from parents to offspring.

germ—Any disease-carrying organism, such as bacteria.

glucose—Form of sugar used as the body's basic energy source; all carbohydrates the body can digest are eventually turned into glucose in the body.

glycogen—The main form in which carbohydrates are stored in the body.

goal setting—Specifying an end or result a person tries to achieve; should be specific, realistic and measurable.

gram—The basic unit of mass and weight in the metric system, equal to about 1/28 of an ounce.

grilled—Cooked on a grill over a heat source.

guidelines—Principles or rules that help determine a course of action.

heart disease—A group of problems that occur when the heart and blood vessels aren't working the way they should.

heart rate—The number of times the heart beats in a set period of time.

heatstroke—A failure of the body's heat-control mechanisms, caused by too much exposure to heat.

high blood pressure—Pressure of the blood against the blood vessel walls that is higher than normal.

hollandaise—A creamy sauce made of butter, egg yolks, lemon juice and other ingredients.

hormone—A chemical secreted by a gland or the brain that signals parts of the body to grow and change.

hydrated—Being supplied with enough water or fluid.

hypothermia—Lower than normal body temperature.

influence—To have an effect on or change someone's thoughts, beliefs or behaviors.

Health Terms Glossary

(continued)

intake—Taking in; the amount taken in.

intense—Very strong; characterized by much action, strong emotion, etc.

intensity—A measure of the level of effort required to perform an activity.

internal—Coming from inside a person.

internal organ—A part inside the body that performs a specific function.

irrational—Not based on facts or reason.

lanugo—A downy growth of soft hair on the body; symptom of anorexia.

laxative—A substance or drug that loosens the bowels to cause bowel movements.

lean—Containing little or no fat.

measurable—Able to be measured or appraised.

media—All the various means of communication used to inform, entertain or influence people; includes advertising, newspapers, radio, magazines, movies, music, music videos, TV shows, websites, computer games, blogs, podcasts and social media.

metabolic rate—The amount of energy released and used from food consumed per unit of time.

metabolism—The process by which the body uses food to release energy and uses the energy to build and repair body tissues.

milligram—One thousandth of a gram.

minerals—Inorganic compounds that play a role in human health.

misperception—An incorrect or false understanding.

moderate—Within reasonable limits; of medium quality, amount, etc.

moderation—Avoidance of extremes.

monitor—To keep track of the condition or progress of something.

muscle tone—Normal, healthy condition of muscles.

negative—Destructive or disruptive.

negative body image—A negative view or dislike of one's body and how it looks.

nutrients—Substances living things need to take in from the environment to live and grow. For the human body these are water, carbohydrates, fats, proteins, vitamins and minerals.

nutrition—The study of diet and health.

nutritionist—A specialist in diet and health.

Health Terms Glossary

osteoporosis—A condition that results from a decline in bone mineral content, which makes bones more likely to break.

peers—People of the same age or close in age who are similar in many ways.

physical activity—Bodily movement that greatly increases energy use.

physical fitness—A set of attributes that add to a person's overall health and physical capability. Some are skill-related (such as balance, agility and speed). Others are health-related (such as cardiorespiratory endurance).

positive—Helpful, constructive or healthy.

positive body image—A positive view, liking or acceptance of one's body and how it looks.

poultry—Domestic fowl, such as chickens, turkeys and ducks.

pressure line—Something said to compel or urge someone to do something.

priorities—Things that are put ahead of other things in order of importance; things given attention before other things.

processed foods—Foods that have been changed from their natural state to make them safer or more convenient.

processed sugar—Sugar usually made from sugar cane or beets that is refined so that it has a regular texture and flavor.

protein—A nutrient made up of carbon, hydrogen, oxygen and nitrogen, whose major function is the growth, maintenance and repair of body tissues.

puberty—Stage of life when the body changes and the reproductive system matures.

purge—To get rid of something, specifically, to attempt to rid the body of food; includes self-induced vomiting and laxative or diuretic abuse.

range of motion—The full distance and direction a joint can move.

realistic—Actually possible, practical.

recommended—Suggested or advised.

refined grain—Grain that has been milled or processed to remove the bran (outer husk) and germ (part that can grow into a new plant) to give it a finer texture.

registered dietitian—A person trained in the study of diet and health who has passed an exam and fulfilled certain requirements.

reliable—Able to be relied upon, dependable.

resisting pressure—Not giving in to the influence or demands of someone else.

responsibilities—The things a person has a duty toward or has made a commitment to do.

© ETR **HEALTH**_Smart_ Middle School

Health Terms Glossary

(continued)

roleplay—An activity in which participants respond to a sample situation and act out roles to practice skills such as resisting pressure or resolving conflict.

saturated fat—A type of fat, usually found in animal sources, that is solid at room temperature. Diets high in saturated fat are linked to greater risk of developing heart disease.

scalloped—Baked with a milk sauce and bread crumbs.

sedentary—Inactive.

self-starvation—Severely restricting calories or depriving oneself of food.

serving—A single portion of food or drink.

snack—A food eaten between meals.

sodium—An alkaline chemical element; in relation to food, usually refers to salts.

specific—Clearly and exactly presented or stated.

strength—The ability of muscle to exert force.

strengthen—To make stronger.

stress—Mental or physical tension or pressure.

sucrose—Sugar taken from sugar cane or sugar beets.

supplement—Something, such as vitamins or herbs, added to the diet, often in the form of a pill or powder.

symptom—Signals the body sends when ill; a condition or effect caused by an illness or disease.

technique—A method of doing something, such as advertising a product.

toxin—A poisonous compound that causes disease.

trans fat—A fat formed by adding hydrogen to liquid fat to make it solid at room temperature; developed to make shipping and storage of foods easier. Trans fats are unhealthy and are linked to increased blood cholesterol levels.

trustworthy—Able to be trusted; worthy of confidence.

type 2 diabetes—A chronic disorder in which the body's use of carbohydrates is impaired, which leads to a deficiency of the hormone insulin. Type 2 diabetes used to be called "adult onset diabetes," but is being seen more often in children and teens. It can often be controlled by diet.

unsaturated fat—Type of fat that doesn't raise blood cholesterol levels.

Health Terms Glossary

(continued)

utensils—Tools or containers, especially those used in the kitchen, such as spoons, forks, knives, etc.

vigorous—Done forcefully or energetically.

virus—An organism formed of genes surrounded by a protein coating; cannot reproduce itself but must invade a living cell to replicate.

vitamins—Organic substances either made by the body or found in foods. Small amounts are essential for the regulation of metabolism and normal growth and functioning of the body.

warm up—To do some gentle movements before physical activity to allow breathing and heart rate to rise gradually and prepare the muscles to use energy efficiently.

weight management—Keeping the body weight at a healthy level using healthy means.